Why I Treat PTSD the Way I Do
Your Seventeenth Psychiatric Consultation
William R. Yee M.D., J.D.
Copyright Applied for 09/16/2020

Introduction
The Pervasiveness of Aggression and PTSD

Attention deficit hyperactivity disorder (ADHD) is a type of developmental disorder, which is characterized by hyperactivity, impulsivity, and inattention.

ADHD affects around 2.5% of the population.

Individuals with ADHD have numerous impairments of cognitive, emotional, and social functioning. And this affects their day-to-day life.

One of the major daily activities, which get affected due to ADHD, is driving.

Individuals with ADHD have been reported to be involved in greater number of driving accidents due to their aggressive behavior and anger. Moreover, ADHD increases the number of traffic violations, associated injuries, and increased chances of dying during a driving accident.

Medications have very limited effectiveness for the treatment of both aggression and Post Traumatic Stress disorder, hereinafter referred to as PTSD.

For deeper consideration of various concepts touched upon in this book I refer the reader to my prior publications:

Assault in Hospitals:
Theory, Policy and Management
Your 5th Psychiatric Consultation
By William R. Yee M.D., J.D.
Copyright Applied for Aug 19, 1983

Self-Mutilation, Suicide, and Homicide:
It is in Your DNA
Your 9th Psychiatric Consultation.
William Yee M.D., J.D.
Copyright Applied for 02/29/2020

The Business of Medicine:

The Patient a Revenue Stream,
The Physician a Tool
Your Sixth Psychiatric Consultation
William Yee M.D., J.D
Copyright Applied for Jan. 11th, 2020

Why I Don't Prescribe Xanax
Or Any Benzodiazepine
Your Sixteenth Psychiatric Consultation
William R. Yee M.D., J.D.
Copyright Applied for 09/13/2020

The Pervasiveness of Aggression and PTSD

Aggression is in fact pervasive over time and across all ethnic groups and cultures. It is found among all primates and is a major force for the progress and chaos of culture among homo sapiens.

Self-mutilation and suicide are a small facet of aggression and explains the concurrence of murder suicide. It is so common that most of it is not reported in the mainstream press except for extreme examples or exceptional circumstances.

Aggression in war, criminal enterprise, and domestic situations is largely operational, i.e., used as a tool, rather than the rare presentation as a product of mental illness.

Not guilty by reason of insanity is a rare occurrence.

"War is a failure of politics," and operational violence.

Homicide is more likely to occur as a sport than a product of mental illness. Serial killers are present in all times and all places and can appear perfectly normal to their neighbors and victims.

Temporary insanity is so rare that it is newsworthy. It is labeled as, "berserk, amok, stir crazy, cabin fever, etc," and manifests as brief agitated homicidal episodes of killing.

Two thirds of adolescents destroy property, make threats of violence, or commit act of violence directed at others during displays of anger.

See:
Epidemiology of juvenile violence
D P Farrington , R Loeber
Child Adolesc Psychiatr Clin N Am. 2000
Oct;9(4):733-48.
PMID: 11005003

About 7.8% of the general population is diagnosed with Intermittent Explosive disorder manifesting with destruction of property, threats of violence or actual violence directed at family, friends, neighbors, peers in school, work, and the community at large. This is often reported in newspapers as road rage or workplace violence. This is particularly true of the developmentally disabled who have few social skills and acquire advantage over more intelligent people with violence.

See:
Intermittent Explosive Disorder in the National Comorbidity Survey Replication Adolescent Supplement
Dr Katie A. McLaughlin, PhD, Dr Jennifer Greif Green, PhD, Irving Hwang, MA, Nancy A. Sampson, BA, Dr Alan M. Zaslavsky, PhD, and Dr Ronald C. Kessler, PhD

Arch Gen Psychiatry. 2012 Nov; 69(11):
1131–1139.
doi: 10.1001/archgenpsychiatry.2012.592
PMCID: PMC3637919
NIHMSID: NIHMS404585
PMID: 22752056

This has a huge impact on the general
population.

Pervasive violence manifests as verbal
aggression, internet and other stalking,
physical, and sexual violence imposed
upon about 36% of women and 33% of men
in the United States. The violence rated as
severe in 21% of US women and 15% of US
men.

See:

Screening for Intimate Partner Violence,
Elder Abuse, and Abuse of Vulnerable
Adults: US Preventive Services Task
Force Final Recommendation Statement
doi:10.1001/jama.2018.14741

The Socialization of Aggression

Having determined that aggression is pervasive, let us examine the patterns of emergence and socialization of aggression.

Every mother is familiar with the "terrible twos." This refers to temper tantrums commonly displayed at about the age of two and the time of potty training.

This is a critical stage in psychosocial development. It is at this stage that the frontal lobe of the brain matures, and executive functions emerge.

The executive functions of the frontal lobe assert control over bowel and bladder spinal cord reflexes.

Executive functions of the frontal lobe grasp and process abstract and complex concepts such as right and wrong, good and bad, and social relationships.

Executive functions of the frontal lobe distinguish between family and stranger.

Executive functions of the frontal lobe master temper or aggression or fail to master aggression and temper.

The executive function of the frontal lobe grasps and processes the concept of the Golden Rule, "treat others the way you want them to treat you."

The executive functions of the frontal lobe grasp and process the behaviors of others to determine if they submit to the Golden Rule.

Failure of the Frontal Lobe Executive Functions to mature during the terrible twos results in antisocial and borderline personality disorders.

Male incontinence ranges from 3% to 11% as overall prevalence of incontinence in the male population. That is a substantial percentage of the population with failure of frontal lobe executive functions maturing over a very basic social function.

See:

The Prevalence of Urinary Incontinence
Victor W Nitti, MD
Rev Urol. 2001; 3(Suppl 1): S2–S6.
PMCID: PMC1476070
PMID: 16985992

Failure of frontal lobe functions to socialize aggression is substantial.

About 3% of the male population and 1% of the female population can be diagnosed with antisocial personality disorders with failure to properly socialize temper and aggression. They are predators that fill prisons, jails and are found in every religion, every ethnic group, and every nook and cranny of organized society.

Borderline personality disorder occurs in about 1% of the population.

The borderline personality disorder has an impaired ability to recognize the needs and feelings of others.

The Borderline personality often presents as a predatory victim, accusing others and demanding unreasonable time, care and attention from friends and relatives.

As a result, the Borderline Personality often burns out all their friends and relatives who eventually refuse to submit to the excessive demands for time, attention, and aid.

The Borderline Personality is very often left alone without the help of any friend and relative who will describe a history of many failed efforts to help without the Borderline Personality helping themselves.

The legal system does not allow antisocial personality disorder to be classified as a mental illness for the purpose of avoiding criminal prosecution.

There are very many borderline personality disorders in jails and prisons because that diagnosis does not excuse criminal activity either.

Although many borderline personalities are the victims of abuse, they are also often involved in allegations of being perpetrators of physical and sexual abuse.

I worked in state psychiatric hospitals where some of the patients made weekly or daily allegations of sexual abuse by staff, even though staff were videotaped sitting in the chair outside of the room while doing one to one supervision for suicidal behaviors.

The borderline personality is the most difficult patient to treat in my opinion. Many psychiatrists refuse to work with borderline personalities in state hospitals, prisons and jails. It can get real ugly real fast.

Self-Organizing Systems

The reader should become familiar with, "Self-Organizing Systems."

I suggest as a starting point the following articles for fundamentals in math and conceptualization.

Advanced Synergetics

Instability Hierarchies of Self-Organizing Systems and Devices
Authors: Haken, Hermann
© 1983

and

Self-organizing individual differences in brain development
Marc D. Lewis University of Toronto, 252 Bloor St. West, Toronto, Ont., Canada M5S 1V6
Received 30 September 2005, Revised 20 October 2005, Available online 13 December 2005.

For this book the issues of stability and instability in self organizing systems are treatment targets for the mental health professional.

I suggest the following as a starting point on the issues of stability and instability.

The importance of dynamic systems approaches for understanding development☆

Author links open overlay panel Mark L. Howe Marc D. Lewisba Lancaster University, Lancaster, UK University of Toronto, Toronto, Canada
Received 27 September 2005, Available online 15 November 2005.

And

I recommend the following because of the extensive Bibliography published online

Self-Organization in Clinical Psychology. In: Hutt A., Haken H. (eds) Synergetics. Encyclopedia of Complexity and Systems Science Series. Springer, New York, NY. Schiepek G., Perlitz V. (2009) https://doi.org/10.1007/978-1-0716-0421-2_472

The notion of self-organizing systems is that they are governed by a few simple rules that allow for prediction of behavior in the near future. However, because the rules are governed by the mathematics of nonlinear equations, prediction fails in the mid and long term.

There is the Butterfly Effect whereby very tiny differences in starting conditions in initial points in time result in very large differences over time.

Well known self-organizing systems are weather, the stock market, politics, war, and any biological or social organization that is governed by such simple rules and nonlinear equations. That includes the growth and development of the brain, the individual from birth to death, the family from marriage to divorce, the neighborhood, the city, the state, any religion, any ethnic group, any species over time.

Common to all the self-organizing systems are periods of stability alternating with periods of chaos.

Biological systems have multiple layers of negative feedback loops encoded in the DNA to maintain stability.

That stability is interrupted by change from both the inside during maturation and aging and from the outside that results in periods of chaos and physical, emotional and behavioral instability.

Examples of change resulting in chaotic instability of emotions and behaviors include the following.

In the individual there are social demands of potty training and control of temper tantrums in the terrible twos.

There is separation anxiety with separation from the family and admission to the classroom and strangers at the age of five.

There are the hormonal changes of puberty and the demands of pairing and sexuality in adolescence.

There is the pruning process in the brain and the demands of independent living in late adolescence and early adult life.

During adult life there are changes in employment, health problems, bankruptcies, divorce, retirement and deaths of friends and relatives.

Failure of the Frontal Lobe Executive Functions to mature during the terrible twos results in antisocial and borderline personality disorders.

Antisocial Personalities have no empathy, have no guilt, have no remorse and feel free to abuse and exploit others. They are predators that fill prisons and jails and are found in every religion, every ethnic group, and every nook and cranny of organized society.

Prior to the age of eighteen the convention is to diagnose antisocial personalities as conduct disorders. At the age of eighteen the convention is to diagnose these same people as antisocial personalities.

I have been physically and verbally abused by this group from the time I entered kindergarten to the present day. I believe that just about everyone that I have met has had the same experience. If you have met a thousand people in your life you have met forty of these people. Your chances of meeting forty of these people without being abused verbally or physically is rather small. This group is very skillful at being abusive and avoiding prosecution and incarceration.

A tiny percentage of incarcerations occur at the time of the first crime.

Borderline personality disorder occurs in about 1% of the population.

The borderline personality disorder has an impaired ability to recognize the needs and feelings of others.

The Borderline personality often presents as a predatory victim, accusing others and demanding unreasonable time, care and attention from friends, relatives, and strangers.

As a result, the Borderline Personality often burns out all their friends and relatives who eventually refuse to submit to the excessive demands for time, attention and aid.

The Borderline Personality is very often left alone without the help of any friend and relative who will describe a history of many failed efforts to help without the Borderline Personality helping themselves.

The treatment of emotional, physical and behavioral instability are invoked with the perception of, "disability," perceived by the parent, patient spouse, teacher, employer or other stakeholder.

What are the diagnosis and treatments of temper tantrums in the terrible twos?

The immature brain with instability of emotions and behaviors may be viewed through many lenses.

There is controversy about bipolar disorder in childhood.

If a child has severe irritability, severe emotional instability, and severe temper outbursts some pediatric psychiatrists will diagnose bipolar disorders.

Others will argue for ADHD, oppositional behaviors, conduct disorder or intermittent explosive disorder, PTSD, or Traumatic Brain Injury.

The subjective face of psychiatry has more weight than the scientific base in child psychiatry.

The recent findings that bipolar disorder can be outgrown in the fourth decade of life would suggest that late maturation of frontal lobe executive functions is misdiagnosed as bipolar disorder.

I offer the following learned treatise for your consideration:

University of Missouri-Columbia. "Young Adults May Outgrow Bipolar Disorder." ScienceDaily. ScienceDaily, 29 September 2009. <www.sciencedaily.com/releases/2009/09/090929141530.htm>.

Rarely does the insurance industry allow for serial Halsted-Reitan neuropsychological evaluations, serial functional magnetic resonance imaging, serial neurohumoral evaluations and extensive and intensive psychotherapy.

In general, these children are subjected to serial medication trials from every class of psychotropic medications including, but not limited to, mood stabilizers, antipsychotics, psychostimulants such as amphetamines, and antidepressants.

Mental illness is not a straight line.

Mental illness is wavy with ups and downs.

If the medication is offered at the peak of the severity of the cycle, the subsequent decay in the severity of the symptoms is mistakenly attributed to the medication.

When the cycle progresses to the next increase in symptoms the medication is increased and as the symptoms cycle down it appears that the medication was again effective.

As this cycle progresses children can find themselves on very high doses of medications.

Examination of adults treated as children will often reveal the diagnosis progressing from ADHD to PTSD, to Depression, to Schizophrenia, to Mania, to Bipolar Disorder and finally to Schizoaffective Disorder.

Often these patients will have a history of being treated with psychostimulants such as amphetamines, anxiolytics such as Ativan, antipsychotics such as Haldol, antidepressants such as Zoloft, and finally mood stabilizers such as Lithium.

Hindsight is 20/20 and an impartial teacher for those willing to learn.

When reviewing these charts since 1972 I have had these thoughts many times.

It appears that the child and family, having weathered the chaotic storms of maturation, have approached a series of psychiatrists.

The psychiatrists walked the patient and family through the PDR in a desperate effort to find the magic bullet that would solve the problem. The psychiatrists left no stone unturned and offered every possible diagnosis along with medications from every class of psychotropic medications.

I have received many of these children in state hospitals after failures by many psychiatrists, many hospitals, and many medications to control their tempers and aggression.

The reality is that children have immature and changing brains. There is failure of the frontal lobe executive functions to control emotions and behaviors.

There is no way to determine if the failure of the frontal lobe is by choice or if the patient is like the color blind and simply unable to see any color except red.

The treatment of mental illness in general and the treatment of PTSD specifically involves meditation, physical exercise, and various psychotherapies, including, but not limited to, Stress Inoculation with Prolonged Exposure, Eye Movement Desensitization, Cognitive Behavior Therapy, Eye Movement Desensitization and Reprocessing, Imaginal Flooding.

The treatment of aggression is such a failure that the legal system does not allow Antisocial Personality to have status as a mental illness.

Prisons solve the problem that psychotherapy and medications cannot solve. Ted Bundy was a serial killer who was executed rather than treated in a mental health diversion program.

The Number Needed to Treat

Medications may be added to treatments listed above, but the failure rate is high, and the benefits are not robust and come with substantial side effects including weight gain, diabetes and numerous other health problems over time.

The single most neglected fact in the practice of psychiatry is the Number Needed to Treat.

Most psychiatric medications require a minimum of at least three or four patients treated with the first medication for one patient to get better.

After the first medication fails the number needed to treat increases to a minimum of four, five or six for one patient to get better.

Each additional trial results in an increase in the number of patients needed to be treated for one patient to get better.

If the patient has had years of treatment under many psychiatrists with many medication trials the prospect of finding a medication that is effective is remote, or very small.

Concurrent with the Number Needed to Treat is the Number Needed to Harm. As the dosage of the medication increases the number of patients needed to be treated to harm becomes smaller and smaller.

Physiologic Reserves and LD50

This is because of the physiologic reserves in the biochemistry of life and the negative feedback loops created by the

DNA to maintain stability and the life of the organism.

The easiest way to understand physiologic reserves is to learn about the LD-50.

The LD-50 is the dose of anything at which half the people die.

The LD-50 for alcohol is a good starting point. Half the people who drink thirteen shots of 40% alcohol, (80 proof), over a short period of time would be expected to die. Some could consume more before dying and some would consume less before dying.

It is very common for young men to encourage each other to drink twenty-one shots on their birthday. Of course, some of them die. This happens at fraternity parties during hazing and probably occurs among young men elsewhere, including among men on active duty in the military.

The LD-50 for water is six liters. Half the people who drink six liters of water over a short period of time would be expected to die. Some could consume more before dying and some would consume less before dying.

The LD-50 for caffeine is 118 cups of caffeine.

Half the people who drink 1,800 mg of caffeine over a short period of time would be expected to die. Some could consume more before dying and some would consume less before dying.

Caffeine can be purchased in pure form on the internet. A teaspoon of pure caffeine has 4706 mg. There are newspaper articles about young men dying from a single teaspoon of caffeine powder or heavy ingestion of caffeine energy drinks.

Let us examine physiologic reserves for chronic low dose exposure to medications.

The physiologic reserves of newborns are very low and increases with age. In middle age the physiologic reserves decline so that the elderly have very low physiologic reserves.

That is why the flu kills the very young and very old more often than young adults.

A young child can die from nicotine toxicity from a cigarette butt, while a young adult can chew on a wad of tobacco all day long while playing baseball.

Tardive Dyskinesia is abnormal motor movements at rest. Tardive dyskinesia is caused by exposure to conventional neuroleptics, anticholinergics, toxins, substances of abuse, and other agents.

Exposure to different medications and chemicals cause destruction of dopamine receptor cells in the basal ganglia, the striato-pallido-nigral system. Destruction of these Dopamine Receptor Cells causes Tardive Dyskinesia.

Although young adults have high physiologic reserves, chronic exposure to conventional neuroleptics, anticholinergics, toxins, substances of abuse, and other agents at low therapeutic doses will destroy the dopamine receptor cells in the basal ganglia, the striato-pallido-nigral system.

Tardive Dyskinesia is also an example of how medical conditions can cause severe reduction in physiologic reserves.

A single dose of conventional neuroleptics, anticholinergics, toxins, substances of abuse, and other agents such as Reglan, (metoclopramide), a dopamine receptor antagonist used for treatment of a variety of gastrointestinal symptoms can cause tardive dyskinesia in young adults with low physiologic reserves.

The populations at risk include, but are not limited to, patients with fetal alcohol syndrome, other developmental disabilities, and other brain disorders.

For this reason, psychiatrists should avoid use of antipsychotic medications for the treatment of the mentally retarded, patients with fetal alcohol syndrome, patient was Traumatic Brain Injuries which are common among active duty military and military personnel discharged with Traumatic Brain Injuries.

I rely on:

Which patients are at highest risk for tardive dyskinesia (TD)?
Updated: Oct 17, 2018
Author: James Robert Brasic, MD, MPH;
Chief Editor: Selim R Benbadis, MD

Patients with Traumatic Brain Injuries are at risk for Sleep Apnea which can be aggravated by sedating medications including antipsychotics and benzodiazepines.

Psychiatrists treating Traumatic Brain Injuries need to become familiar with the treatment of organic insomnia, fatigue, narcolepsy (with and without cataplexy), sleep apnea (obstructive and/or central), periodic limb movement disorder, parasomnias, depression, anxiety and pain.

I rely on:
Traumatic Brain Injury and Sleep
Disorders
Mari Viola-Saltzman, D.O. and Nathaniel
F. Watson, M.D., M.Sc.

The Case Against Benzodiazepines

Respiratory Arrest and death are greatly
increased when diazepines are added to
opiates or the elderly with sleep apnea.

The VA is now treated elderly veterans
from World War II, Korea and Vietnam, as
well as Iraq and Afghanistan.

PTSD and Traumatic Brain Injuries are
the major issues faced by the psychiatrist
treating active-duty military and VA
patients.

Because Schizophrenia emerges in late
adolescence and early adult life it is also a
serious issue affecting active-duty
military personnel.

The intersection of Post-Traumatic Stress
Disorder, Traumatic Brain Injury,
Schizophrenia, and drug addiction and

abuse are difficult, and treatment failures are high, as measured against the standard of a functional recovery.

The long-term use of addicting medication is generally contraindicated for the mentally ill.

I rely on:

Benzodiazepines Tied to a 41% Increased Mortality Risk in AD
Batya Swift Yasgur, MA, LSW
November 28, 2017

The chronic use of benzodiazepines is known to increase the death rate of the mentally ill.

I rely on:

Mortality of Patients Dependent on Benzodiazepines
B Piesiur-Strehlow, U Strehlow, W Poser
Acta Psychiatr Scand 986 Mar;73(3):330-5.
Doi
10.1111/j.1600-0447.1986.tb02693.x.
PMID: 3716850 DOI: 10.1111/j.1600-0447.1986.tb02693.x

Benzodiazepines increase the death rate of patients with schizophrenia.

I rely on:
Polypharmacy with Antipsychotics, Antidepressants, or Benzodiazepines and Mortality in Schizophrenia
Jari Tiihonen, MD, PhD; Jaana T. Suokas, MD,
PhD; Jaana M. Suvisaari, MD, PhD; et al,
Jari Haukka, PhD; Pasi Korhonen, PhD
Arch Gen Psychiatry. 2012;69(5):476-483.
doi:10.1001/archgenpsychiatry.2011.1532

The use of benzodiazepines and sleeping pills increase mortality by 40% to 60%.

I rely on:

Mortality associated with anxiolytic and hypnotic drugs—A systematic review and meta-analysis
Ajay K Parsaik, Soniya S Mascarenhas, Darrow Khosh-Chashm,
First Published November 20, 2015,
https://doi.org/10.1177/0004867415616695

It takes two to four years for medical statistics to be compiled for publication.

Even though benzodiazepines tend to make mental illness worse, mental illness was the primary reason for prescribing benzos such as Xanax.

Even though combining benzodiazepines such as Xanax with opioids can result in fatal respiratory arrest, benzodiazepines are prescribed with an opioid medication one third of the time.

I rely on:

Office Visits at Which Benzodiazepines Were Prescribed: Findings From 2014–2016 National Ambulatory Medical Care Survey by Loredana Santo, M.D., M.P.H., Pinyao Rui, M.P.H., and Jill J. Ashman, Ph.D.
National Health Statistics Reports Number 137
January 17, 2020, U.S. DEPARTMENT OF HEALTH AND HUMAN SERVICES
Centers for Disease Control and Prevention National Center for Health Statistics Physician

Kaiser Permanente and the VA have policies against the use of Benzodiazepines for the treatment of Post-Traumatic Stress disorder.

I rely on:

Benzodiazepine and Z-Drug Safety Guideline
Kaiser Permanente
Last guideline approval: January 2019

And

VA » Health Care » PTSD: National Center for PTSD » Providers » Treatment » Use of Benzodiazepines for PTSD in Veterans Affairs

More than twelve percent of the United States population (12.6%) are prescribed benzodiazepines every year. It appears that the trend is for increasing use of benzodiazepines.

I rely on:
Benzodiazepine Dependence, Toxicity, and Abuse: A Task Force Report of the.

The Treatment of Active Military Personnel

The military accepts men and women into active duty starting at the age of eighteen. I have met patients who submitted false documentation and were able to enter active duty at the age of fifteen.

These young men and women are faced with rigors of basic training, separation from family, and exposure to extreme violence, while also dealing with the following:

There are the hormonal changes of puberty and the demands of pairing and sexuality in adolescence and young adult life

There is the pruning process in the brain.

There are traumatic brain and other injuries experienced during active combat.

Traumatic Brain Syndrome and diffuse brain damage from pathological pruning during late adolescence and early adult life share anosognosia.

Anosognosia is the lack of awareness of parts of self, including awareness of body parts, emotional parts, sensory inputs, memories, imagination of thoughts, and sensory inputs including hot, could, pain, numbness, past, present, and future possibilities.

I rely in part on:

What Neurological Syndromes Can Tell Us about Human Nature: Some Lessons from Phantom Limbs, Capgras Syndrome, and Anosognosia
V.S. Ramachandran
Cold Spring Harb Symp Quant Biol 1996. 61: 115-134
doi:10.1101/SQB.1996.061.01.015

Traumatic brain injuries are a common result of injuries from improvised explosive devices, or IED's.

During childhood the brain has a broad array of potential skills that are honed with play and studies.

During adolescence there is pathological pruning of neurons that are not used.

It is believed that pathological pruning can be caused by inflammation, viral infections, chemical exposures, use of drugs, and possibly traumatic brain injury.

It is also believed that brain pruning of unused neurons is a lifelong process.

In general, it is believed that every 100 days the brain fingerprint changes by 13%. That thirteen percent is where the effect of psychotherapy and other treatments of Traumatic Brain Injury, Schizophrenia and PTSD can be measured directly on an empirical basis.

The 87% of the brain fingerprint that does not change controls the vegetative and sensory functions and stable portions of the personality that do not change in response to stress, psychotherapy and medications.

I rely on:

Dietrich College of Humanities and Social Sciences
November 15, 2016
Researchers Develop Way To "Fingerprint" the Brain
New Tool Uncovers How Brain's Structural Connections Are Individually Unique
Contact: Shilo Rea at 412-268-6094
Dietrich College of Humanities and Social Sciences
5000 Forbes Avenue, Pittsburgh, PA 15213
(412) 268-2830
Legal Infowww.cmu.edu

Treatment of Schizophrenia in the Military

Approximately 250,000 military are recruited every year with the average enlistment age of average enlistment age of just under 21.

The United States will allow enlistment of a seventeen-year-old teenager into their military with parental consent and eighteen-year-old without that consent.

One of my cousins joined the military at age seventeen with a promise that she would not be sent to Iraq until she was eighteen. My aunt was very angry when she was sent to Iraq at the age of seventeen. She completed her tour of duty and was given an honorable discharge. She is doing well

The age of onset of schizophrenia is late adolescent and early twenties for males and a slightly older age for females.

Newly enlisted military recruits are at risk for schizophrenia.

Age of Onset of Schizophrenia: Perspectives From Structural Neuroimaging Studies
Nitin Gogtay, Nora S. Vyas, Renee Testa, Stephen J. Wood, and Christos Pantelis
Schizophr Bull. 2011 May; 37(3): 504–513.
doi: 10.1093/schbul/sbr030
PMCID: PMC3080674

PMID: 21505117

The goal of treating new recruits with first onset schizophrenia is a functional recovery.

The pharmaceutical industry and the medical literature warn of a functional decline with each acute psychotic break and recommend maintenance doses of antipsychotic medications once started.

The maintenance doses invite weight gain, diabetes, tardive dyskinesia, gynecomastia, galactorrhea and a host of side effects over time.

However, Thomas R. Insel, M.D, Director of the National Institute of Mental Health (NIMH) from 2002-2015, points out the fact that after the initial psychotic break patients who stop antipsychotic medications achieve a functional recovery at the rate of 40.4 percent after seven years.

He adds that after the first psychotic break patients who continue antipsychotic medications for the next seven years achieve a functional recovery of only 17.6 percent after seven years.

Patients with schizophrenia who are treated without maintenance antipsychotic medications achieve more than double the rate of functional recovery compared to those who are treated with maintenance antipsychotic medications.

I rely on:

"Post by Former NIMH Director Thomas Insel: Antipsychotics: Taking the Long View," By Thomas Insel on August 28, 2013.

In psychiatry the best practice is the lowest effective dose.

My experience in psychiatry since 1972 is that if patients don't respond to low doses of antipsychotic medications, they are not likely to respond to high doses of antipsychotics or polypharmacy.

I treat mental illness. I do not cure mental illness.

As early as 1956 it was determined that a single dose of 100mg of Thorazine or 25 mg of Thorazine three or four times a day is sufficient to resolve the psychosis of Acute Intermittent Porphyria.

I rely on:

September 15, 1956
CHLORPROMAZINE IN THE TREATMENT OF PORPHYRIA
James C. Melby, M.D.; John P. Street, M.D.; C. J. Watson, M.D.
JAMA. 1956;162(3):174-178.
doi:10.1001/jama.1956.02970200022005

Thorazine does not cure Acute Intermittent Porphyria.

It is not known by what mechanism Acute Intermittent Porphyria causes psychotic episodes that respond to Thorazine.

It is speculated that because Thorazine binds to the D_2 dopamine receptors, the antipsychotic effect is due to blockade of the D_2 dopamine receptors.

It is believed that hallucinations, delusions and paranoia of schizophrenia are due to hyperactivity of dopamine at D_2 dopamine receptors in the mesolimbic pathway of the brain. Thorazine binds to those receptors.

D_2 stimulators (agonists) include opiates, alcohol, nicotine, amphetamines, and cocaine. The use of opiates, alcohol, amphetamines, and cocaine is associated with psychotic episodes and aggression.

It is speculated that the flat affect, lack of psychosocial motivation and engagement, and other negative symptoms of schizophrenia may be due to under stimulation of the D_1 receptors.

What is the optimum dose of an antipsychotic medication when used in the treatment of schizophrenia?

A study demonstrated that from two to five milligrams of haldol a day achieved 60% to 80% saturation of the D_2 receptors in the brain.

That same study revealed that blood levels of 0.51 ng/ml of haldol achieve 50% D2 occupancy and blood levels of 2.0ng/ml of haldol achieves 80% D2 Occupancy

There was a dispute as to whether 70% or 90% D2 occupancy is necessary for adequate therapeutic effect.

I rely on the following:

Kapur S1, Zipursky R, Roy P, Jones C, Remington G, Reed K, Houle S.
Psychopharmacology (Burl). 1997 May;131(2):148-52.

In 2000 research determined that 0.02 mg/kg/sc of haloperidol achieves 50% saturation of D2 receptors. For a two-hundred-pound man that is 2mg achieves 50% saturation.

I rely on:

Dopamine D 2 receptor blockade by haloperidol.
Kapur S1, Barsoum SC, Seeman P.
Neuropsychopharmacology. 2000 Nov;23(5):595-8.

Research has determined that
1-65% D2 saturation by Haldol achieved a therapeutic response,
2-72% saturation by Haldol raised prolactin levels and
3-78% saturation by Haldol precipitated extrapyramidal side effects.

Not all the patients responded to Haldol.

When the patients who responded to haldol were examined it was determined that there was:
1-no relationship between saturation above 65% and clinical response.
2-That is raising saturation above 65% did not appear to yield additional benefit.
3-raising D2 saturation above 65% increased prolactin levels and extrapyramidal side effects.
4-2.5mg a day of Haldol achieved 65% to 75% D2 occupancy.
5-The recommended Haldol starting dose was 2 or 3 milligrams a day.

I rely on:
Relationship Between Dopamine D $_2$ Occupancy, Clinical Response, and Side

Effects: A Double-Blind PET Study of First-Episode Schizophrenia Shitij Kapur, M.D., Ph.D., F.R.C.P.C., Robert Zipursky, M.D., F.R.C.P.C., Corey Jones, B.A., Gary Remington, M.D., Ph.D., F.R.C.P.C., and Sylvain Houle, M.D., Ph.D., F.R.C.P.C. Am J Psychiatry 157:4, April 2000

Clinician and family are advised to treat with the equivalent of 100mg of Thorazine and monitor Prolactin Levels. If the prolactin levels are normal the risk of Tardive Dyskinesia is low. There is little benefit from increasing the dose beyond the 100mg equivalent of Thorazine to justify acquiring Tardive dyskinesia.

To assist in the use of low dose treatment of schizophrenia it is useful to have the following Thorazine Equivalency Table

First generation antipsychotic medications:

Chlorpromazine Thorazine..... 100mg
Fluphenazine Prolixin............ 2mg
Haloperidol Haldol................ 2mg
Loxapine Loxitane................ 10mg
Perphenazine Trilafon........... 8mg

Pimozide Orap...................... 2mg
Prochlorperazine Compazine.. 15mg
Trifluoperazine Stelazine........ 2.5mg
Thioridazine Mellaril............. 100mg
Thiothixene Navane.............. 4mg

Second generation antipsychotic medications:

Aripiprazole Abilify................ 7.5mg
Asenapine Saphris................. 4mg
Clozapine Clozaril 100mg
Iloperidone Fanapt 3.5mg
Lurasidone Latuda................... 16mg
Olanzapine Zyprexa................. 5mg
Paliperidone Invega 2mg
Risperidone Risperdal.............. 1mg
Ziprasidone Geodon 60m

There are many Thorazine Equivalent Charts available online and the reader is advised to fact check before using my chart as there may have been updates and I may have typographical errors.

Summary of Treatment of PTSD, TBI, Schizophrenia Among Soldiers

When I started practicing psychiatry, I offered psychoanalysis and individual psychotherapy in addition to medications.

I performed physical examinations when I admitted patients to the hospital for treatment.

I ordered all manner of laboratory tests and consultations with specialists.

I practiced medicine through the lens of psychiatry.

With the evolution of medical insurance and the interventions of MBAs to control costs I find that currently the primary care physician authorizes lab testing, consultations and special treatments.

I find that I am limited to prescribing medications and social workers, psychologists and psychiatric technicians now offer psychotherapies.

For the treatment of PTSD
benzodiazepines should be avoided.

The only justification for their use is in
the emergency room or a psychiatric
hospital when a patient is agitated,
violent and in need of immediate sedation
for safety reasons.

The primary treatment of PTSD should
not be medications.

The primary treatment of PTSD should be
meditation, physical exercise, and various
psychotherapies, including, but not
limited to, Stress Inoculation with
Prolonged Exposure, Eye Movement
Desensitization, Cognitive Behavior
Therapy, Eye Movement Desensitization
and Reprocessing, Imaginal Flooding.

For the treatment of first episode
schizophrenia low dose antipsychotics
should be used only for the acute
psychotic break.

After resolution of that psychotic break
maintenance antipsychotics should not be
used to maximize functional recovery.

If maintenance antipsychotic medications are necessary, the active-duty patient is not likely to recover sufficiently to continue active-duty assignments.

That is because of the rigors of military duty and the high level of physical and mental performance necessary to complete assignments.

For traumatic brain injuries benzodiazepines and antipsychotics are generally not effective and are contraindicated.

Mood stabilizers should be managed by neurologists who should be the team leaders in managing traumatic brain injuries.

William R. Yee M.D., J.D.
Board Certified Psychiatrist.
Practicing Medicine and Psychiatry without
interruption since 1972 in Michigan, Indiana,
Kentucky and California.

Recently licensed in Texas and excited about
opportunities to live and practice in Texas, at
your service.

"Pre-Existing text," includes names of symptoms, medical illnesses, medications, people, corporations, law cases, statues, text of statutes, the titles of articles, of books, the content of articles and books cited.

My copyright claim is a clam to the "original text," which is my personal experiences as described in the text above and my commentary on the names of symptoms, medical illnesses, medications, people, corporations, law cases, statues, text of statutes, the titles of articles, of books, the content of articles and books cited.

www.ingramcontent.com/pod-product-compliance
Lightning Source LLC
Chambersburg PA
CBHW021930170526
45157CB00005B/2257